The Ultimate Guide To A Fast:

Metabolism

Finally Get In Shape, Lose Weight And Make Your Metabolism A Weight Loss Machine!

I0417009

Chris Smith

STOP!!! Before you read any further....Would you like to know the Secrets of Body Transformation?

If your answer is yes, then you are not alone. Thousands of people are looking for the secret to rapidly burn body fat, keep the weight off, become healthier, and truly transform their body and life for good.

If you have been searching for these answers without much luck, you are in the right place!

Not only will you gain incredible insight in this book, but because I want to make sure to give you as much value as possible, right now for a limited time you can get full **100% FREE access to a VIP bonus EBook** entitled **THE 7 KEYS TO BODY TRANSFORMATION!**

<u>**Just Go Here For Free Instant Access:**</u>

www.liveFitVIP.com

Legal Notice

Disclaimer Notice

Table Of Contents

Introduction

I want to thank you and congratulate you for purchasing the book, "Metabolism: The Ultimate Guide To A Fast Metabolism! - Finally Get In Shape, Lose Weight And Make Your Metabolism A Weight Loss Machine!"

This book contains proven steps and strategies on how to get the body you have always wanted, but even better still you will have the health to go along with it.

If you are reading this then most likely you haven't reached your goals yet, but in your heart you know you deserve to be in the best shape of your life. Don't worry, unfortunately society has made it much harder to lose weight than it actually is.

When you have the right formula losing fat or building muscle is really no different than baking a cake. You put the right amount of ingredients in, at the right time, and viola you have a perfect looking cake that tastes good too!

But in contrast to the perfect cake, if you are missing one ingredient you will have a much different outcome! Getting in shape, whether you are trying to build muscle or lose fat is much the same. All you have to do is follow a good recipe to the T and you will end up with an amazing looking and healthy body!

If you are looking for sound principles that can get you lean, muscular, and healthy, then look no further! Read this book, apply these principles and you will find that not only do you look incredible, but you feel amazing, healthy, and full of energy.

Thanks again for purchasing this book, I hope you enjoy it!

Chapter 1 – Health And Its Importance

"Health is the First wealth."

I remember the first time I heard the saying *"Health is the First Wealth"*, I was at the gym actually, in the middle of a hard workout, feeling frustrated that I hadn't reached my goals yet. Then I saw a poster, that seriously looked like it was from the 80's that had a guy on it that was in ok shape, sweaty with a bottle of water, you know the kind. Anyways, I read this saying, *"Health is the First Wealth"* and thought to myself - "Why is health the first wealth? Isn't it being in shape?!"

Well, as you get older you do start to appreciate the saying. Health truly is the first wealth. Because at the end of the day, what really matters is that you can have a functional body that allows you to enjoy your life with friends and family doing the things that make you happy! But the really good news is this. If you do it right, not only will you create a healthy body on the inside, but you will also create an incredibly sexy looking body on the outside! So let's remember first and foremost how lucky we are to be healthy! And if you aren't currently healthy, then use the desire for health to fuel your ambition for reaching your goals.

You want to look good but you also want to feel incredible! Why have a healthy looking body, without a healthy body? The good news is working to make sure that you are healthy on the inside will help you achieve the look you want on the outside. In other words, you need a plan that will create a lean body on the outside and an overall feeling of well-being and health on the inside.

Physical Health

A healthy body receives good nutrition, and has regular physical activity, and ample rest. This is so important because if you miss one of these ingredients, you will most likely also be lacking in the other areas.

Alright now that we have that out of the way let's get started!

Chapter 2 – Metabolism & How Calories Are Burned

Metabolism:

Everyone knows that the key to fat loss and losing weight in general is to have a fast metabolism. So why are we all so mystified by the ever illusive metabolism?

I'm sure you remember hearing someone either joyously stating that they can eat whatever they want, or on the other hand, stating how they can't eat something because they have a slow metabolism. The good news is this book is going to help take the mystery out of metabolism and more importantly how you can crank yours up!

When a person aims to lose weight, one of the things people usually state is "how many calories can I eat". Most people are almost a slave to this number, and feel very constricted when they hear that they can eat X amount of calories if they want to lose weight.

But there is a trick! I'm going to let you in on a little secret that many bodybuilders know and use to their full advantage. For every pound of muscle you build on your body, you automatically burn about 50 more calories per day!

So let's say you are able to pile on 10 pounds of muscle. Now is the time where you are saying, but, but, but, I don't wanna gain weight I wanna lose weight!

Ok I know, but bear with me here. Let's say you are able to put on 10 pounds of quality lean muscle, meaning no extra fat, just solid muscle. Those 10 pounds are going to actually burn an extra 500 calories per day just to remain on your body, but the trick is you have to keep exercising them if you want to keep them.

Now that you know this important detail, how important do you think building muscle is if you want to lose fat? Pretty darn important! So the key to creating a faster metabolism is building lean muscle!

Definition

Calories are units of energy. In terms of everyday language and in nutrition, calories pertain to the consumption of energy through eating and drinking. It also refers to the usage of energy through various physical activities. A calorie is actually a unit of heat energy. Calories are acquired from carbohydrates, fat and protein.

So in more plain English, calories are needed for energy. Sometimes the calories we expend are from the food we have eaten recently, and sometimes the calories come from stored glycogen and fat on our bodies. Sometimes the calories we burn come from muscle on our bodies. It all depends on how you eat and workout which determines where the calories come from.

Calories are in food and drinks; anything that has energy actually has calories. The body recognizes calories as energy, and it's the energy needed to produce heat. Heat energy is what actually fuels the body – it's comparable to gasoline needed by cars to run and function.

How Many Calories Are Needed to Lose Weight?

Every person has a different daily calorie requirement. The ideal calorie consumption depends on various factors, which include physical activity, overall health, weight, height, sex and body shape. If you want a leaner body, you just have to make sure that you spend more calories than what you consume.

Case in point: a soccer player may need more calories than a 75-year old woman.

Health organizations are still undecided as to what the average person's ideal calorie consumption is: some say men require as much as 2,700 calories each day, and women require 2,200, but for some, they say it should be around 2,500 and 2,000 respectively.

The United Nations, on the other hand, believes an average adult should consume at least 1,800 calories a day.

This is actually quite ridiculous if you think about it. How can you set a generic amount of calories for every man or every women? In truth finding the right amount of calories for you to achieve the body you desire requires much trial and error on your part. This book will give you a good idea on where to start, but it is up to you to tweak the calories up or down until you achieve the ideal bodyweight and fat composition.

There are three major factors involved in calorie calculations:

- Physical activity

This includes everything from making the bed in the morning, jogging, walking, and those activities that involved moving around. The number of calories burned in the said activities depends on your body weight.

- Basal metabolic rate

    This is the amount of energy needed by the body to function even at rest. This also includes the required energy needed by bodily functions (this keeps your heart beating, eyelids blinking, lungs breathing, and body temperature stabilizing). I highly recommend going online and searching "Basal Metabolic Rate Calculator". You will find many of these free calculators. I would do a few of them so that you can derive an average. This calculator will tell you how many calories you body burns just resting without exercise. This gives you a baseline to understand how many calories you will burn in a day.

- Thermal effects of food

    This is the energy used in digesting the food you eat; the energy is required to process the breakdown of food down to the basic elements that the body needs to use. This is where it can get interesting because it actually takes more energy to burn certain types of foods than others. My advice on this is to just think about it logically. If you put a piece of meat outside on your driveway and left it there, and you also put a piece of moist cake next to the meat on the driveway, which food would you expect to stay there longer. Imagine how long would it take for the cake to be destroyed in a heavy hail storm or snow storm? Probably not very long. On the other hand, the meat would most likely last through many storms as it is much tougher and dense.

Well this is kind of how it works in your body. It requires very little energy for the body to burn or to break down a piece of cake that has very little density. But the meat takes a lot of energy for the body to burn it and digest it, because it has to break down the dense strong fibers of the food.

What you need to take away from this chapter is this. Losing fat and gaining muscle is a process. In order to lose fat, the body should receive fewer calories and you should engage in more physical activities such as cardio routines. If you want to build muscle, then you will need more calories than the body burns. But keep in mind what type of foods you put in, because they do burn at different rates. What really is important is to know that if you want to be able to eat more, you need to put on lean muscle in addition to trying to lose fat.

Chapter 3 – The Healthy Fat Burning Diet

It's easy to eat, but it's hard to eat smart. Find out how a balanced diet not only helps you lose those unwanted pounds, but also keep you healthy in general.

A funny thing about people and fitness goals is they often tell themselves some type of story. Everyone does it. Either you tell yourself that you don't like this type of food or you only can eat this way...etc...etc...etc. But the truth of the matter is anyone can change if they put their mind to it, if they have a good enough purpose for making the change, and lastly if they have a plan of action and they actually follow it.

What is a Healthy Diet?

A healthy diet helps improve or maintain your general health. This type of diet gives your body the essential nutrition that it needs: enough amino acids from protein, enough fluids, enough vitamins, minerals, fatty acids, and calories.

Having a healthy diet does not mean that you should starve yourself; it is not about adhering to strict principles either such as completely removing specific food types. It's about having more energy, stabilizing your moods, feeling great, and keeping yourself as fit and healthy as possible.

What Foods Make Up a Balanced Diet?

For the body to function properly, it needs to have essential nutrients. Eating healthily means you'll eat a balanced diet consisting of a food variety with the right amounts. A balanced diet contains various types of foods to give you all the nutrients required.

Which foods (or food groups) make up a balanced and healthy diet?

- **Whole Grains** – These provide your body with vitamins, minerals and fiber. According to experts, the recommended intake should be three ounces daily. This is where many people get into trouble. Three ounces is not much, but many people like to make whole grains a major staple of their diet, when in actuality they should just be a small portion of the overall diet. It is recommended that you eat unrefined cereals, breads and pasta made of whole grains.
- **Fruits and Vegetables** – One of the best eating habits that can be implemented is the regular intake of fruits and vegetables. This should also be your diet's cornerstone. This will help prevent the development of various dangerous diseases such as cancer, type 2diabetes and heart disease. If you want to go wild with anything in your diet, it should be with vegetables! Try to eat lots of vegetables as they are not only very low in calories, but fill you up better than any other food source, and to top it off are amazingly healthy!
- **Protein** – Protein comes from poultry, meat, beans, eggs, soy, nuts and fish. Protein is necessary to repair and build

tissues. Protein should definitely be a staple in your diet, as it takes the body much energy to burn and it also aids in building muscle.

- **Dairy Products** – Eating dairy products won't always make you fat so long as you keep track of the fat content. Dairy products keep your bones strong, and these products include yogurt, milk and cottage cheese.
- **Legumes** – Legumes help in preventing diseases such as type 2 diabetes and heart diseases. Legumes include clovers, lentils, soy and beans.

The take home - It's best to have all these foods included in your daily diet. Just shoot for the proper proportions of each of them.

Chapter 4 - Eating For Metabolism

Any diet can be used to get the lean body you want, but the key is you should not be depraving yourself and feeling like you are starving; it should be about eating the right portions of nutrients for your goals spaced out in equal sized nutritious meals.

In order to have a healthy diet, you don't have to stop eating or to deprive yourself of foods that you love. Moderation is the key. Your goal should be to develop a diet that can be maintained for life, not just because you're aiming to lose weight in the short term. The principle behind eating for metabolism is to eat healthy, nutritious foods that assist in building muscle and losing fat.

The following is a discussion on the right amounts of nutrients needed for a healthy and fit body

Carbohydrates

It is said that carbohydrates should comprise around 30-60% of your diet, depending on the level of physical activities you engage in. The more active you are, the higher your carbohydrate requirements. It's because carbohydrates are needed for energy – it helps you lift heavier weights, and perform repeated exercise sets to continually gain muscle.

If you lack carbohydrates in your body, your body may burn your existing muscles or use the protein from the food you eat – this will make it hard for you to build and repair tissues, which means that it would be difficult to gain and maintain muscle mass.

Here are the types of carbs you should eat, and the type you should avoid.

- **Healthy Carbs** – these include beans, fruits, whole grains, and vegetables. These carbs are digested slowly which makes you feel full longer. These carbs also keep insulin and blood sugar levels stable.
- **Unhealthy Carbs** – these include refined sugar, white flour and white rice that have been removed of fiber, bran and nutrients. These digest quickly as well as cause spikes in energy and blood sugar levels.

Protein

It is said protein should make up 25-50% of your diet. Muscles are made up of water and protein; for every pound you weigh, you should eat ½ to 1 ½ grams of protein. This is necessary for your body to repair and rebuild your muscles and make them stronger.

Protein gives the body the energy to get up and keep going. The protein stored in food is broken down into 20 amino acids needed for the maintenance of cells, tissues and organs. Amino acids are also the body's building blocks for energy and growth.

Just remember that eating too much protein won't help you gain muscles faster; any excess protein will just be used for energy or building fat. Eating to Little protein on the other hand will slow down the growth of your muscles.

Fats

Fats should not be avoided completely; in fact it is said that fats should make up around 10-20% of your diet. Fats are necessary so your body can produce muscle building hormones such as testosterone.

Good resources of healthy fat help nourish your heart, brain and cells, as well as your skin, hair and nails. It's important to eat foods rich in omega-3 fats called DHA and EPA because they can reduce the chances of acquiring heart diseases, improve moods and help avoid dementia.

Add the following to your diet:

- Omega-3 and Omega-6 fatty acids – these are found in fatty fish like herring, salmon, anchovies, sardines, mackerel, and some supplements of cold water fish oil. Other sources also include corn, unheated sunflower, flaxseed oils, soybean and walnuts.

- Monounsaturated fats that come from plant oils: olive oil, canola oil and peanut oil, as well as avocados, seeds (sesame & pumpkin) and nuts (hazelnuts, almonds and pecans).

On the other hand, avoid or at least reduce intake of these fat types:

- Trans fats which are found in processed foods made with partly hydrogenated vegetable oils, vegetable shortenings, crackers, some margarines, cookies, candies, fried foods, snack foods, and even baked foods.

- Saturated fats which are found mainly in animal sources; these include whole milk dairy products and red meat.

Water and its Role towards a Better Body

Aside from oxygen, water is the second most important substance to maintain life. The body is made up of 50-70% water. Without water intake, the body can only survive for up to 3-4 days. Metabolic processes, especially those related in the synthesis of nutrients for burning fat and building muscles require water supply.

The amount of water needed daily is related to the person's metabolic rate. It's also dependent on parameters such as level of physical activity and weight.

Here's the rule of thumb in drinking water: for every 45 pounds weighed, a liter of water should be drank every day. Therefore, a person who weighs 160 pounds should be drinking about 3.5 liters of water each day.

A lot of people find it difficult to drink the required amount of water intake. It could be that you're just not thirsty, or you just forget to drink. Here are tips on how it can be easier to meet your daily water intake requirements:

- Start early. Drink your first liter of water in the morning; this makes it easier to meet the recommended daily amount.
- Eat food with high water content. Fruits and vegetables could contain water too, so it's ideal to eat them on a regular basis. Not only would doing so enable you to meet water intake requirement; it also allows you to meet your vitamin requirements.

- Water should always be available. Have a glass or bottle within reach, whether you're at home, at work, or on the road. Drink from your
- containers regularly, even with small sips. Refill the container once it's empty.
- Drink water with each meal, as well as during and after training and workouts.

Chapter 5 – Exercising To Boost Metabolism & Gain Muscle

If your goal is to lose fat and to get lean, then you need to create a big enough calorie deficit to lose the fat and to see a difference in your body.

For you to lose one pound in a week, a 3,500 calorie deficit should be created, i.e. you should burn 3,500 more calories than the amount of calories taken from the food you eat.

An ideal exercise routine should take about 45 minutes – a mix of strength training and cardio exercises – and should be about six times a week. Sweating is not necessary, but the burned calories need to add up for it to matter.

Cardio Exercises

Cardio exercises should be an essential part of a weight loss program. Cardio exercises get your heart pumping and can burn fat in various intervals in relation to the workout's intensity. If you indulge in low intensity cardio, you'll build stamina better, while short rounds of high intensity exercise will burn more calories and maximize fat loss. It could improve your metabolism for the long-term. You may have to perform cardio exercises five to six days per week though if you have a lot of fat to burn.

Weight Training Exercises

In general, the ideal program to achieve a lean body should focus on exercises using large muscles and make use of short rest periods. As previously mentioned, the best trainings are those which are a mix of heavy training and cardio.

Weight training would not only improve strength; it would also help build muscle. The growth of muscle tissue is only stimulated when there is pressure on it. You may do reps from time to time, but if you use light weights, your muscle will not receive the necessary pressure; hence, your muscles will not respond and grow.

Another beneficial weight workout is about doing more reps using moderate weights. This routine is beneficial because the muscle fibers used are 'slow-twitch', which means they hold less glycogen, and so less glycogen will be removed from the body during these workouts. This is needed to keep building muscles and to enhance metabolism.

The Importance of Rest

If you think all you need is a proper nutrition and an effective workout routine, then think again. The best diet,   training program and even a supplement routine will not be as effective if you do not get enough rest – and getting enough sleep is the best way to achieve that

Rest and recovery is a vital part of building muscle tissue. During sleep, you produce growth hormones, and protein synthesis takes place.

What are the other important sleep functions?

- During sleep, the body has lower energy consumption. To conserve body resources, the body uses lowered energy consumption as a biological mechanism. If you don't have enough sleep, then your body would compensate by requiring many meals each day.

- Sleep repairs muscle and other tissues; it also replaces dead and aging cells.

- Sleep recharges the brain. Levels of adenosine (powers the cells' biochemical reactions) decline during sleep which suggest that during sleep, the brain is refreshed. When the brain rests, the body benefits because mental alertness is needed during the day, especially when training.

Sleep is important, especially for body builders; it restores brain functions and gives you alertness. It also helps prepare for intense training sessions. Having enough sleep – ideally 8-10 hours every night, also helps in enhancing muscular recovery through human growth hormone releases and protein synthesis.

Chapter 6 – The Whole Package Fitness & Health

A healthy lifestyle will leave you energetic and keep you away from diseases. This type of living will depend on the choices you make and your everyday habits. It is about accountability and taking responsibility for your actions and decisions that will affect your body for the present and the future.

It's never too late to adopt a healthy lifestyle. You can always start a healthy life regardless of age, body shape or fitness level.

If you feel you don't live healthy enough, then you can always begin today. It doesn't matter if it's just baby steps, as long as you're moving towards a better life ahead.

Benefits of a Healthy Lifestyle

A healthy lifestyle is an important – if not the only – way to reduce the chances of health issues, recovery, coping with stress and improving the quality of life.

Scientific evidence shows that lifestyle plays a huge part in a person's health – from the food you eat, the exercise you do, whether you drink, smoke, or do illegal drugs; it all affects your health, not only affecting how long you'll live, but how long you'll live without having chronic diseases.

Better lifestyle habits minimize your chances of illnesses such as heart conditions. You'll feel better and more energized. It also improves your moods, and helps you feel happy and confident. Not only do you get to live longer; you also get to experience a better quality of life.

Components of a Healthy Lifestyle

A healthy lifestyle is made up of components necessary for a better life. How do you stack up on the list?

Physical Health

Physical health pertains to how the body functions. Fitness should be a major factor in your life. Physical fitness helps you get better sleep, keeps your weight in check, prevents health problems such as stroke, and makes your life longer in general.

Exercising has a lot of benefits; your life won't really be complete without it. You may also want to avoid alcohol abuse for obvious reasons.

Environmental Health

This is about how you keep your surroundings clean – your air and water, as well as your food. It's also about keeping your surroundings safe and enjoyable.

Social Health

Social health refers to how you maintain your relationships with your family, friends and loved ones, as well as your teachers and classmates; these are basically the people you hang around and interact with.

Spiritual Health

Spiritual health is all about the maintenance of a harmonious relationship with other people, animals and other living things; this is also about having purpose and spiritual direction. This is also about living according to one's morals, values and ethics.

Mental / Intellectual Health

This is the ability to cope with daily life's demands as well as the capability of recognizing reality.

Emotional Health

Emotional health is all about expressing your feelings and emotions in a positive and non-destructive way.

The previously mentioned health components all affect one another; if one of those is weak, it can possibly affect your overall health. You can always choose what your actions are that will make you move either closer or farther from optimal health.

Maintaining Your Body

Achieving a healthy body is good, but learning how to maintain it is even better. A person only has one body throughout his lifetime; it's best to understand how he can take care of it in the best way possible. So how can you maintain a healthy body?

Understand how your body can be harmed. It's one thing to know the things that can be beneficial to your body; knowing what can harm it is another.

Three factors can affect the body in a major way: malnutrition, injuries and microorganisms. As long as you understand how these can be prevented, then you can be safer.

Just Keep Going. The lifestyle changes you have implemented to achieve that leaner body should be an ongoing process. The best thing about achieving the lean physique you want is that you may not need to work out as rigorously as before. Once your metabolism is improved, it will be easier to manage weight. You will also appreciate how great you feel and it will be much easier to motivate yourself to stay fit.

Conclusion

Thank you again for purchasing this book on boosting your Metabolism through quality nutrition and exercise!

I hope this book was able to help you to understand and implement the principles of getting lean, muscular, and healthy. You can never be comfortable living a life that is unhealthy. I have dedicated myself to educating you on how to lose fat the healthy way.

The next step is to get started on becoming who you dream to be! Also, if you know of someone else that could benefit from the information in this book, please tell them about it.

Finally, if you enjoyed this book, please take the time to share your thoughts and post a review on Amazon. It'd be greatly appreciated!

Thank you and good luck!

Preview Of:

<u>Intermittent Fasting Diet</u>

Lose Fat in 7 Days Intermittent Fasting!

Introduction

I want to thank you and congratulate you for purchasing the book, "Intermittent Fasting Diet - Lose Fat in 7 Days Intermittent Fasting!".

This book contains proven steps and strategies on how Intermittent Fasting can not only help you lose fat rapidly, but keep it off for life!

Have you been working out consistently? Eating the recommended 4-6 meals each day? And still, you are unable to reveal your six pack and glutes to the world?

You are not alone. For years supplement companies, fitness magazines, bodybuilders, fitness trainers, health gurus, and many others have been all telling the same advice to lose fat and gain muscle. Their solution for your fitness goals - Eat 4-6 miniature chipmunk sized meals, do lots of weight training, and even more cardio. So, the time is now to ask yourself one simple question, "How's that working out for ya?".

If you don't feel too good about your fitness results, and really want to see that six pack, lean muscular physique, then you are reading the right book. The time is now to try the most revolutionary new diet, which I would rather refer to as a lifestyle - Intermittent Fasting!

Thanks again for purchasing this book, I hope you enjoy it!

Chapter 1 - Intermittent Fasting And Its Benefits

Intermittent fasting is markedly different from any other diet plan that you may have tried in the past. Most weight loss plans espoused by fitness gurus will tell you to control the amount you eat while keeping a close watch on the kinds of food that you do consume, usually in combination with a rigorous exercise routine. You know this: you've done the cardio, lifted the weights, run the miles, and eaten 6 small meals a day, all the while assiduously avoiding unhealthy fats and unnecessary carbohydrates.

But you are probably reading this book because this system just doesn't work for you – in fact, it has probably left you tired, crabby, and frustrated, with nothing to show for your hard work but a few insignificant inches shed from your waistline and some mad food cravings that are proving harder and harder to ignore.

This is not to say that typical diet programs don't work. After all, there's a reason why they have their staunch advocates. But the fact remains that for most people, it is much more effective – and much easier – to control when they eat, instead of what they eat and the portions thereof.

That's what intermittent fasting, also known as IF, is all about. To put it in the very simplest terms, when you adopt this lifestyle, you will only eat during a certain period of time daily, and go entirely without food, which is the fasting bit for the rest of the day. That's all there is to it. And, once you consider the amount of time that there actually is between meals, you'll see that it isn't hard at all.

There is no denying that exercise and healthy eating are important (you can't hope to get that six-pack if you live on fast food burgers and stay on the couch all day, but more on that later), but intermittent fasting can work wonders on its own. Before we go on to the nitty-gritty of this fitness lifestyle, let's take a look at the unique benefits that it has to offer.

Better Weight Control and Faster Fat Loss

Since shedding pounds and losing inches are the most conspicuous signs of success of any diet program – not to mention your most likely objective when you start dieting –we'll start here. Intermittent fasting is exceptionally effective at helping you lose fat since it eases your body into a situation where it starts burning fat stores for energy. And since this will happen every single day that you go through a period of fasting, you will lose fat faster and have better control over your body weight than if you stick to counting calories.

Elimination of Pesky Food Cravings

One of the major trials for any dieter is the craving for snacks and sweets, and, admittedly, those will still be there when you start intermittent fasting. Once you get into the habit, however, you'll find that your pesky food cravings aren't troubling you as much, and soon you just won't feel them anymore. Scientists theorize that this is due to fasting bringing the level of your body's ghrelin, otherwise known as the "hunger hormone", down to normal, so you don't continually feel the urge to snack.

Reduced Oxidation with Boosted Autophagy

Oxidative stress caused by free radicals in your system can really take its toll on your body's cells. The damage done by free radicals to DNA, RNA, proteins, and lipids is known to advance the effects of aging and disease. Going on an intermittent fasting diet will help combat this by boosting autophagy, or the process by which cellular waste is recycled by your body. This helps your cells get rid of the trash, so to speak, so that they can continue to function optimally, allowing you to better withstand stress, disease, and aging.

A Healthier Nervous System and Mental Clarity

Though it is commonly believed that fasting will leave you weak and unable to think, nothing could be further from the truth. Intermittent fasting has actually been shown to enhance memory and learning, as well as helping to improve your disposition in life. This is because periodic fasting boosts the production of brain-derived neurotrophic factor (BDNF), a hormone that prevents the degradation of the neurons in your brain while stimulating the growth of new neurons. A boost in the neurotransmitter serotonin also happens, which leads to better moods and improved learning ability.

Enjoyable Longevity

While any sort of health and fitness regime has the long-term aim of prolonging your life, one of the main attractions of intermittent fasting for many people is that it promotes enjoyable longevity. Good health shouldn't mean giving up good food, or spending the rest of your long life obsessively counting calories. Intermittent fasting is a lifestyle that allows you to eat the way you like (up to a point!) while staying fit. In addition to that, scientific studies have shown that fasting can increase an animal's lifespan without retarding their growth, which is not the case for diets that focus on caloric restriction.

Thanks For Previewing My Exciting Book Entitled:

"Intermittent Fasting Diet: Lose Fat In 7Days Intermittent Fasting"

To purchase this book, simply go to the Amazon Kindle store and simply search:

"INTERMITTENT FASTING DIET"

Then just scroll down until you see my book. You will know it is mine because you will see my name "Chris Smith" underneath the title.

Alternatively, you can visit my author page on Amazon to see this book and other work I have done. Thanks so much, and please don't forget your free bonuses

DON'T LEAVE YET! - CHECK OUT YOUR FREE BONUS BELOW!

Free Bonus Offer: Get Free Access To The www.LiveFitVIP.com VIP Newsletter!

Once you enter your email address you will immediately get free access to this awesome newsletter!

But wait, right now if you join now for free you will also get free access to the "The 7 Keys To Body Transformation" free EBook!

To claim both your FREE VIP NEWSLETTER MEMBERSHIP and your FREE BONUS EBook on THE 7 KEYS TO BODY TRANSFORMATION!

Just Go To:

www.liveFitVIP.com

www.ingramcontent.com/pod-product-compliance
Lightning Source LLC
Chambersburg PA
CBHW070937290526
45795CB00003B/1049